The Virus and The Vaccine:
A Story of Deception

Tyler Lazarus Stump /
Mister. E

ISBN
Fonts by Me. Thank You.
Printed, Distributed and Bound in the United States of America First Printing
September 2022
Published by He Who Rebels Against All
Oklahoma City, Oklahoma 73106

Hey, Thanks for getting a copy!
Facebook.com/TylerLazarus1992
Facebook.com/Oddityler

I have an entire bestselling series dedicated to these events.
It's called 'KONG FLU PANDA'
BASED OFF THE 1968 HONG KONG FLU PANDEMIC.

I WOULD LOVE FOR YOU ....to check them out.

The Virus and The Vaccine:
A Story of Deception

Tyler Lazarus Stump / Mister. E

LAB NOTES:

LAB NOTES:

WUHAN WARNING:

In 2020, the first act of global bioterrorism, and biowarfare began.

It employed a SARS Bioweapon against Human Biological Systems.

It was created because of lax bioethics, biosecurity and biocontainment procedures. The gates of Rome were down, and the invaders didn't come in barbarian costumes, but bat costumes.

And things, soon become batshit.

It spreads as an epidemic. It becomes a pandemic within two months.

The entire world enters into lockdown within 90 days.

Within 5 months, 300,000 are dead.

Within just 2 years, 6-23 million die. Isolated in hospital wards, and alone.

It originates in Wuhan, China.

1,000 feet away from The Wuhan Institute of Virology.

An institute of Virology which had been receiving over
30 million dollars in grant funding.
Specifically, American Funding.

Tens of millions die,
From tens of millions of dollars – all designed to do it.

The paper trail, in tens of millions of dollars, is
initially denied.
In both actuality and plausibility.
They scoff at it as an impossibility.
"Not us" The Chinese Scientists Say.
Then, within a few months, an internal leak of
financial receipts are revealed.

The paper trail, and the money trail goes back directly
to the National Institute of Health.

And one Anthony Fauci.

Authorizing said funding.

The Nation's (America's) top immunologist. The most
celebrated disease specialist.

--- has been quietly helping to create deadly
pathogens by administrative approval and
authorization.

And also endorsing Chines Communist Bioweapons

programs, with direct ties to CCP bio-defense contracts.

No surprise, in his own words, he once stated the sentiment "that if another pandemic happened, the resulting information gained from it would be worth it."

He meant the resulting loss of life. When you strip away the euphemisms, and word play he loves to engage in. He means death. Intentional. Pre-meditated.

Back on the ground, hundreds of thousands have now been murdered and fallen suddenly dead to this novel virus.

It spreads radically, beyond even the rate of measles and anthrax.

And it's lethal, in it's first wild, original WUHAN strain.

It becomes weaker, overtime, as it spreads across the map, but never stops being highly infectious.

It starts killing, thousands + thousands a day, at it's peak.

The world completely changes. Almost overnight.

Social distancing, masks, and more measures come

into play.

None of them work. The damage the pathogen creates becomes immeasurable.

None of them slow the pathogen, none of them stop the pathogen.

All preventative measures fail. They prevent neither the spread or the transmission of this engineered virus.

One of the many reasons for this is because it can spread asymptomatically. And invisibly.

Many people wont know they're infected, for some time, before it becomes the disease form with noticeable signs.

It's a silent killer.

And it doesn't only kill people,

It devastates the economic system, the medical system, the political system and continues ravaging and cleverly burrowing inside the human system.

Before detonating.

In a bomb of symptoms and side effects.

You see, it's a lab-enhanced SARS pathogen, but it does MUCH more then create Severe Acute

Respiratory Syndrome.

The breathing and lung problems are the tip of the soon-to-be ventilator iceberg.

It can spread to every human organ and it also crosses through the blood brain barrier.

Some patients EVEN experience psychosis, upon and during infection; psychosomatic illness that presents itself so severely as brain inflammation and encephalitis that some end up committing suicide – because of a total loss of reality. It causes major signal disruption inside the brain and neurological pathways. Horribly.

What this engineered bioweapon does leaves the world at a loss for words.

But, I have a few more of my own.

Chapter 2
While others are shocked, many even shell shocked, even more shocks continue to light up the global sky: Millions.... start dying, quickly.

While a perfect immunological inflammation storm is happening,
another perfect storm is also taking place.

'Coronavirus' becomes a household name, because almost every household in the world eventually ends up becoming infected by it and either surviving it, and being bodily injured, or flat out totally dying from it.

But where did this VIRUS come from?

Certainly not from an Institute of ...VIROLOGY?????

Bioethics News

Bioethics.Georgetown.Edu

"Inside the Chinese Lab Poised to Study The World's Most Dangerous Pathogens."

February 22 2017

"A laboratory in Wuhan is on the cusp of being cleared to work with the world's most dangerous pathogens. The move has generated much excitement as well as some real concerns. Some scientists, outside of China, worry about pathogens escaping, and the addition of a biological dimension to geopolitical tensions between China and other nations."

One Year Later.

The Washington Post

2018

<u>State department Cables warned of safety issues at
Wuhan Lab studying Bat Coronaviruses</u>

"U.S. Embassy officials visited a Chinese research
facility in the city of Wuhan, several times, and sent
two official warnings back to Washington about
inadequate safety at the lab which was conducting
risky studies on coronaviruses... The first cable warns
of the lab's work on coronaviruses and their potential
for human transmission and represented a risk of a
new SARS-like pandemic."

Those Official State Cables end up being totally
ignored. Buried under another stack of paperwork.

Two Years Later.

<u>A Coronavirus Outbreak in the City of Wuhan.</u>

"Global Health Research and Policy"

"The Novel coronavirus outbreak in Wuhan, China

By Hengbo Zhu, Li Wei, and Ping Niu.

and the rest becomes history.

But we're not done with THIS story.

As the pathogen/Bioweapon begins to spread,
China denies all accountability (of course) and by all
accounts, according to them, this just came from their
local wetmarket.

They blame it on food.

The problem with this, is two fold, one: the virus holds
inserts, nucleotides and amino acids that nature will
never bestow upon it.

If the problem was with bad meat, people would be
shitting themselves, everywhere.
Contaminated meat spreads through digestive and fecal
pathways.

Not respiratory and Lung tissue. Not endothelial and
vascular.

Two and most importantly, China has been
SPECIFICALLY working on weaponizing SARS and
Coronaviruses since 2004, as part of their ambitions in
modernizing their Biotechnology and Military
capability.
Military Reports FROM BEIJING even speak on being
able to use Coronaviridae (Coronaviruses) In a new
way to seed global disruption.

Three, not listed, but equally as important for pure
epidemiological conceit:

The virus holds a totally unique furin cleavage site and
the actual spike protein has been greatly enhanced to
evade immunity in the ORF8 protein.

It's been designed – instead of spreading to other
animals as a natural zoonotic, animal based virus
would – to infect the Human ACE-2 receptor cells.

It's been modulated, manipulated and revved up, many
times any natural viruses ability (SARS or other) to
spread, infect, hurt and kill.

It's a murder weapon.

It's a bioweapon.

Blind bats in a cave do not possess the ability to
downregulate the immune system and evade highly
specific immune cells, that only can be created by

playing around and dicking around in a fancy laboratory, to do it.

But people are dicks and they lie, is that truth really a shocking surprise...

To Anyone?

Meanwhile, Every+One is now having to deal with this unleashed monstrosity.

Hospitals −across the world− nearly collapse.

Beds full, Vents used, Nurses quitting right and left because of the pressure and strain to keep so many people alive, all at once.

3 million die within the year.

Hundreds of Millions soon are infected.

And then, re−infected.

The Pathogen spreads and seeds itself across the world map

A Germ, Germinating.

The virus mutates and evolves at a hasty rate and the pandemic moves in waves.

On that same wavelength, you have fingers pointing in all directions, as fatigue turns to hopelessness turns to anger, and you begin to see middle fingers.

The middle class is totally destroyed, financially, at this point.

Business after Business goes under.

Small business, suffering immensely. Gone, overnight.

As you can imagine. Lockdowns, Shutdowns and Deadworkers and constantly hospitalized staff means you cant keep your little job running.

China keeps lying, as countries flounder.

The health agency inside the United States and the Lead Health Advisor and Disease specialist, with the million dollar grants connected to the lab – where it all started – also continues lying.

And why wouldn't he.

He was tasked with preventing disease, NOT helping to cause it.

But he has a sordid history of lying, so a few more wont hurt, not at this point.

It'll hurt tens of millions, but it won't hurt his shady reputation.

People begin to defend the man who funded research to kill them.

Gotta love America.

They'll protect Judas, while he's selling them out and getting his bag of silver.

Outside of films and Tom Clancy Literature, Biowarfare was a term of fiction. Bioweapons, a plot device for spy movies and James Bond scores.

Until it happened in actuality and real, real, reality.

People – lost their minds and lost their shit – and lost their jobs,

And lost their health, their ability to breathe, and then lost their lives.

Such is as a Bioweapon is and does.

When you see a gun, you might think, OII that might be used to hurt people.

Traditional Warfare, and the means in which it employs, are visible, bloody, and even dramatic.

Biowarfare, still uses lethal weapons, but it's a bioweapon = and they aren't visible, they are kill by internally wounding, and people just drop dead.

Biowarfare employs the total reverse of Traditional Warfare but its arguably much more dangerous.

A gun can kill 15.
A modified pathogen can kill 15 million.

Only outside atomic escalation and agency can those numbers be reached by Traditional Warfare.

And the thing is, Biological war leaves the wealth of nations intact, while nuclear warfare destroys everything, both human and the systems in which those humans lived and built.

Biological warfare leaves the city in place.

But all the people, inside that city, dead.

And speaking OF people:

People, for the most part, can AND should be forgiven for their behavioral shortcomings, at the INITIAL phase of the pandemic.

What can't be forgiven is the people that purposefully did this, created this, and unleashed this.

And even worse,

What they do, after, is unforgivable, to themselves and
to others.

Enter The Vaccine.

The Virus and the Vaccine,
A Story of Corruption

Vaccine Technology, synthesized from Biotechnology, which in itself, combines chemistry, biochemistry with biology and THEN pharmacology, is the single–most important tool humans have in the fight to eradicate dangerous disease and harmful pathogens.

But it is a technology, with all of those aforementioned disciplines that DOES require discipline.

In that complicated dance of pharmaceutical creation, drug interactions can become overwhelmingly negative AND fatal, should they go wrong.

Medicine can become Bad Medicine, Instantly.

That product must interact with human cells and tissues, and if that interaction should go awry, you will have millions hurt and possibly killed.

As a side effect.
Of that bad medicine.
Created by bad science and deployed by bad judgement.

For those reasons, THE HIGHEST safety and health measures must be used in stringent doses along with common sense and years of data to ENSURE those things cant and DONT happen.

Unfortunately, they did.

Vaccines that have been studied and undergone the required safety and clinical trials, which take 5-10 years to perform.

TAKE THEM.

Rushed, Mystery Serums made in 4 months with no long term studies or long term data.

Please.
Avoid.

Real vaccines save lives.

Rushed injections will put your life AT risk.

Especially rushed injections made by Felony
Companies.
Companies with the largest felony count on their
record ... in all of medical history.... for creating
previous bad products.

They were.... somehow.... foolishly.... unbelievably....
allowed to manufacture a highly critical and sensitive
new vaccine....
and not just a regular vaccine... a vaccine that deployed
MRNA technology..... the singular most important and
the DEEPEST intercellular tissue process inside YOU
when it comes to protein synthesis..... and that same
felony company was allowed to create this highly
experimental shot...... a product that had never been
taken to market....before.

They were given the full clearance.
REALLY?????????????????........

Yes.

Really.

This REALLY happened.

In the fallout of millions suddenly dying,

the hospital system collapsing, the social system in panic, the economic system crashing, and the human biological system being under siege, en masse,

It's easy to see why calmer heads didn't prevail.

Foolish, politically bereft heads... did.

Enter a supposed savior. *Bright, White Light and Angelic Noises* WAAHHHHHHH

HERE IS THAT SAVIOR:

Dressed as Jesus.

Cosplaying, badly, as Jesus.

But I, Tyler LAZARUS Stump, recognized them as Judas, in disguise.

Right off the bat. As this modified Bat virus was spinning across the map.

These felony companies, all of them, were given the green light to begin starting production of this "vaccine" before regulation was even added to see if It

ACTUALLY COULD VACCINATE.

This was a major red flag.

and it should have been a huge yellow light.

And allowing a company with felony counts for
product fraud....
should have been an INSTANT RED LIGHT.

If actual adults had been in charge.

But, none were.

And so fools charged in.

Where angels fear to tread.

Enter Stroke Victims and Blood Clot Amputation
Survivors.

Within a few months, mass cases of thrombocytopenia,
heart failure, myocarditis, brain bleeds, and
neurological disorders began to appear.

Many of them becoming.... not all surprisingly...

FATAL.

Because Medicine can BE bad medicine, when performed wrong.

To take, imbibe, inject, swallow or inoculate a bad product equals a horribly bad time. With bad, even horrific consequence.

Many people start dying, from the vaccine; the very product meant to save them.

Which, in an even worse turn, of already bad turns, the shot cant even vaccinate. It fails to stop the spread of the virus, it fails to neutralize it, and boosting antibodies fails to even stop death or hospitalization FROM the virus.

And then, the shot begins injuring.

In rapid-fire, shotgun explosion levels. Across the map.

'Sudden Death,' becomes a common buzzword.

Previously healthy 20-30 year olds, begin dropping like flies.

Everywhere.

Heart Attacks, Cardiac Arrests, Strokes, Ischemic

Events, followed by life altering blood clots that require amputation.

The damage from the bioweapon had been severe,

The damage from the rushed shot, maybe even worse.

Tens of millions, maybe upwards to 30 million are now gone to their grave because OF both.

Negatively impacting them, the ones they love, and the entire world.

And the world keeps turning.

Within a week, a social media group called "Suddenly dead News" hits over 300 thousand members. With flood after flood of first hand reports of people losing family members, and people at their jobs, from all of these complications + more. It becomes impossible to hide.

Everyone is noticing what's happening.

Big government and Big media, followed by Big Pharmaceutical try and sweep it under the rug,

Which just ends up amounting to Big Trouble.

Enter The Chaos, Of An Engineered Viral Weapon
and the Fallout of a Destructive, Dangerous and Failed
mRNA Vaccine.

During all of this, which essentially amounts to a
horror movie, happening in slow-motion,

One American President launches an attack against the
US Capitol Building,

Flees, Let's America Implode,

Another president is elected, who then crashes the
country into the ground at 400mph,

Republican + Democrat - both insufferable and highly
annoying - begin to collapse the country AFTER said
national trainwreck, and infighting amongst
themselves.

Two compromised Presidents, One former, One
Current, Both with ties to Russia and China....

AS.... Hilariously Enough,

Russia AND China begin to move in and flex.

Russia invades Ukraine, during this bioweapon

happening,
and China begins licking it's already pathogen-covered
latex glove fingers.

As the West begins to self-destruct, the powers that be
from the East begin to assert dominance, as the world
populace is powerless to obstruct or stop the chain of
events set in motion, by the turning of every MINOR
event leading to the eventuality of one MAJOR
historical transformation.

The Map of power is being redrawn.

America, in all of its star-spangled bravado, will not be
able to sing of the rockets red glare and the bombs
bursting in air, in the same way again, because those
rockets and those bombs flying in the air, might just
be nuclear warheads ----- Flying 10,000 mph -----
headed, directly our way.

As OF this report, America is in a bad position, The
World is severely weakened, people are suddenly
dying, every hour of every day, from the broken and
forced "vaccine,"

And everyday gets worse.

Rome 2.0 is certainly on Fire.

And this time, it's a slow burn,

<u>and a slow crawl to hell.</u>